Home Doctor:
20 Easy Ways How To Use Alternative Medicine To Stay Healthy Without Pills

Table of content

Introduction

There you are, standing in the supermarket once more, trying to find something that will relieve that headache you feel. You have battled this headache for days now, and you are beginning to worry that it is going to turn into a migraine.

Obviously, you are doing what you can to alleviate the pain. You are staying away from loud noises, you are staying away from bright lights. You are staying away from caffeine and alcohol, and you are staying away from refined white sugar.

But, your headache persists. So, there you are, trying to find some sort of relief so you can get out there and function in the real world once more.

But you flip over the box, and you see something you don't like. A long list of side effects that sound terrible. You don't want to put something in your body that has all of those nasty side effects, but it sees the more you turn over these boxes, the nastier side effects you find.

So what do you do?

"I can't go on with a headache like this. I need to have some sort of relief."

"I just want to feel better. I don't know how that's going to happen, but I can't let it go any longer."

"I want to feel better and get back to living the life I'm used to, but I don't want to risk these side effects."

If you have ever felt anything like this, you are not alone. So many people want to avoid dealing with side effects and synthetic medication, but so few people know that you can actually treat yourself with all natural remedies that are just as effective if not more effective than the synthetic pills you find in stores.

And I am going to show you exactly how to use this alternative medicine in your life.

You are going to fall in love with the results, and love the lack of side effects as well.

Let me show you a new way to do medicine, and change the life you live.

Chapter 1 – Getting Started with Alternative Medicine

When it comes to alternative medicine, it's going to take some getting used to for you to go from the way you once lived your life, to the way you are going to live your life now.

Trust me, it's not an overnight transformation, and it's something that is going to take you a while to get used to. More than likely you are going to run into people who do not believe in the uses of this kind of medication, and you almost certainly are going to run into some criticism for doing it.

But, there's a reason alternative medicine has stayed around even through the turns of all the modern medical discoveries... and that is because it works. Sure, there are some things that you are going to have to use synthetic medication for, but all in all, you are going to find that alternative medicine is the way to go.

Which brings us to the first lesson in this book:

Lesson 1. Let go of your view of modern medicine, and open your mind to the alternatives

As you enter the world of alternative medicine, you are going to run into all kinds of people who criticize and doubt how well it works. You have to just let these people have their opinions and stick with what you know.

Of course, do your research and know that you have to do to get through whatever illness you have, but believe in the alternative medication, and have confidence that it really will work for what you need.

It does take some time, and part of it does come through experience, but trust me, it doesn't take long before you see how well it really does work for you. Granted, your faith in this kind of medication is going to grow the more you see it work, but part of that is going to have to come when no one else thinks it will.

What's important is that you stick with it, and see the results for yourself.

This brings us to the second lesson in alternative medicine... you have to know what you are dealing with, and how to treat it.

Lesson 2. Understand what you have and how to take care of it

As you know, if you go into the doctor, they run all kinds of tests, poking and prodding you to determine exactly what is wrong with you so they best know how to treat it.

When it comes to alternative medicine, you may not know the technical term of what you have, but you can know to an extent what it is.

What I mean is… you can know that you have a sore throat, and rule out it being strep throat by looking at the symptoms. If you merely have a sore throat, you are going to treat it differently than if you have something more serious.

This is going to save you both time and money in the doctor's office, but it is going to require you to do a bit of research on your own.

Lesson 3. Learn how to do the research you need, so you know how to treat the symptoms you have

More often than not, you are getting medication to treat the symptoms you are feeling. You aren't necessarily getting medicine to get rid of the illness per se (though sometimes this is definitely the case), but you are actually getting pills to alleviate some of the symptoms you are feeling.

For example:

If you have a cold, you get cold medicine. There's nothing that can cure the cold… it's going to have to run its course. But, the medication you take is going to help with the symptoms you are feeling, making the cold easier to deal with.

So, for lesson three, you need to learn about what you are feeling, and how you can treat these symptoms naturally.

The best way you can do this is to take to the internet. There are hundreds of credible sources that are going to give you list after list of things that will work for the symptoms you are feeling, you just have to take the time to look it up.

Lesson 4. Learn where to source the remedies you find

Now, it won't take you long to realize there are tons of remedies for tons of ailments online, but you aren't necessarily going to find those remedies where you live.

One of the drawbacks to all-natural alternative medicine is that you are somewhat limited by what you have on hand, or in the local stores. Sure, you can order them, but more often than not you are going to end up with some sort of pill if you do things this way, and we already know that's what you are trying to avoid.

So, when you look up the remedies, take the time to also search which ones can be found locally. You may be surprised at what they keep on hand in your local produce section at the supermarket.

Which naturally, brings up the question... organic or non organic?

When it comes to treating ailments through natural remedies, I recommend you use organic as much as possible. This is because you are going to want to stay away from the pesticides that are often used with the non organic produce.

In addition, with all of the GMO foods available on the market today, you will want the added assurance of knowing the remedies you choose are not genetically modified.

Of course, if you only have the choice of pills or non organics, go with the produce instead. Using these is going to be a step up from using the pills, even if you don't have the option of using organic products.

Chapter 2 – The Good and the Bad

It seems no matter what subject you are studying, you are going to have opposing views. Sometimes, these views are so varied they are actual opposites, which can leave you feeling a little confused.

How can you find one source that says this particular remedy works, then find another source that not only says the remedy doesn't work, but that you shouldn't ever use it?

Well that's the world of the internet.

Unfortunately, you are going to have to sift through all the varying opinions if you want to find what really works, and part of that is going to be through a level of trial and error.

Lesson 5. Use sources combined with experience

Obviously, when you are first getting a feel for all natural remedies, you are going to have to read up on each one to decide if that's what you want to use for yourself.

But, you are also going to have to experience some of the things yourself if you are going to make educated decisions in the future.

What I mean by this is that you can't always stand by a remedy if you haven't tried it, because there really are some things that may work for you when they don't work for anyone else, and there are things that may not work for you though you find article after article that swears by it.

The best way to handle things like this is to give yourself a trial basis, and see how you are feeling. If you try something and you don't it, try something else. Or, if you try something and you find that it works great, write it down for future reference.

Lesson 6. Keep your mind open... always

Even in the world of alternative medicine, there are still new discoveries being made. Sure, there are countless sources that stand by what people have been doing for hundreds of years, but at the same time, that doesn't mean you may not run into something new.

There are countless scientists and doctors out there who are still greatly involved with alternative medicine, and they are working to make new discoveries daily.

Make sure you keep an open mind with everything, and that you are willing to set aside an opinion you may have formed for a new way of doing things... all naturally of course.

Lesson 7. Beware of the gimmicks

Every field in life has people who are only in it for the money, and alternative medicine is no different.

If you hear something that sounds too good to be true, odds are, it is. In other words, there is no root that is going to make you lose a hundred pounds doing nothing. There's no miracle oil that's going to give you princess like skin after a single use.

Even in the world of alternative medicine, you have to watch out for those that just want to get a hold of your money. Use your head, and if you hear something that sounds outlandish, it probably is.

Lesson 8. Don't be afraid to talk to professionals

Along with your wariness of those that are just after your money, you do have to remember that there are a lot of professionals out there who are avid participants in alternative medicine.

Depending on what you are treating, you may find that there are local professionals around you who know how to treat or even cure what you are dealing with, and this can be done through a wide variety of treatments.

What is important is that you find the one that works for you, and you go with that. When it comes to the world of alternative medicine, you are going to find that remedies are as diverse as the people who stand by them, and what works for you could take a little while to find.

Enjoy the process and do your research, you will get what you need.

Chapter 3 – Getting to Know Your Options (and How Your Body Responds)

One of the biggest problems with pills is that you only have one option when it comes to treatment: Take the pill.

Of course, when and how you take said pill is varied, but you don't really have any other option besides popping it in your mouth with a glass of water. Sometimes you take the pill with a meal, sometimes you take it first thing in the morning.

However you take it, your only remedy is to take the pill and hope for the best.

Now, when it comes to alternative medicine, you can treat any ailment you have through a range of methods, including ways that don't require you to eat anything.

In fact, you can use these remedies whenever you want and usually wherever you want. The greatest benefit that comes from the use of alternative medication is that you can find what works for you.

Lesson 9. Learn what your other options are

You may have heard of sound therapy, or massage therapy, or acupuncture. These and countless other forms of therapy like these don't require you to eat anything.

You simply massage various points in your body, or you prick your skin with needles (a professional will do this to ensure that it is done right), or you listen to sound waves that are meant to soothe and comfort the soul.

Of course, whether these will work for you depends on what you are treating at the time, but it is good to know what you do have options besides always looking to the pills or produce department.

Lesson 10. Learn the range of treatment options for the ailment you are treating

Just as there are no identical ailments, there's not always a single, black and white method used to treat these ailments. When it comes to how you treat yourself, you need to decide what works for you and how you are going to use it.

Perhaps you do like to eat or sip on something... that's great! There's options. Perhaps you would rather do something more physical. Again, go for it! You have options.

Lesson 11. Listen to your body

With the options you have open to you, it may be tempting to ignore how your body is responding to the treatment.

This can make it difficult to treat yourself, because you have to know when you need to try something else, and how long you need to give something to work. You see, some things do require a little while to build up in your system before they are going to give you the benefits you are after, but at the same time, if something isn't working for you, don't be afraid to try something else, too.

Lesson 12. Stay aware of what you are using, and how they are interacting with each other

When it comes to all natural remedies, you don't have to worry so much about the side effects, because there rarely is anything dangerous or as extensive as what you find in the store manufactured medication.

But, that doesn't mean there aren't any side effects, and you do have to be aware of what you are doing.

For example:

Apple cider vinegar is used for a wide range of ailments, but it's highly acidic. This means that it's going to have adverse side effects if you use too much of it. Monitor how you are feeling while you use your treatment, and you will be just fine.

All in all, if you feel worse by taking a treatment than you did when you started, or if you happen to notice other things happening besides what you were initially feeling, try switching it up.

As I have already said, you are going to find a number of different remedies for a single ailment, so you do have your options.

Chapter 4 – Alternative Medicine with a Mission

One of the biggest mistakes people make when they are using alternative medicine is that they don't give it a chance to work. More often than not, you are going to find a lot of people who tell you it's not going to work, and as a result they aren't sure it is working for them.

This leads to them thinking that there's something wrong with the method they are using, and as a result, they give up on it too soon. I don't want that to happen with you. I want you to get the results you want, and I want you to know without a doubt that it is working for you.

But, part of that is going to be you giving it a chance to work, and you recording how you feel based on the alternative method you are using.

Lesson 13. Give your alternative remedy a chance to work, and actually take note of how well it is working

We have all been in the doctor's office and heard them tell us that we need to give the medication a test run, and if it doesn't work, then we are going to try something else.

You know that if they are going to suggest that with the modern medicine, then of course it's only natural to assume the same with the alternative medicine. The best course of action is to try something, and if it doesn't work, try something else.

If you are feeling something... say, you have a headache... try typing into a search engine 'natural remedies for a headache', and you will be given several different methods to choose from.

This is going to give you the freedom to try one thing, and see if it works. If it doesn't, move on down the list.

Or, you can skim the list and find the methods you like best before you begin, then try those. Another major benefit that comes from the use of alternative medicine is that you are free to use it as you wish, when you wish.

Think of it as the ultimate freedom when it comes to taking care of your health. You really can't go wrong with that.

Lesson 14. Create a list of 'go to' remedies that you can grab whenever you need... it's going to cut down on the time you spend searching for the remedy

As you get better at this, you are going to learn what works and what doesn't, and you can even put together a list of things that do work well for you.

If you keep some of these things on hand, you are going to be set whenever an ailment strikes, eliminating the need for you to go out to the store when you aren't feeling well.

If you are going to put together a wellness box such as this, I recommend you put things in the box that aren't going to go bad. Some of the natural things you can use tend to expire after a shorter length of time than the things that are synthetic, so you are going to have to be choosy when it comes to what you keep on hand.

Of course, if you keep up on your box, you aren't ever going to have an issue with what's getting old.

All in all, find the system that works for you, and you are going to be set.

Lesson 15. Decide what fits your standard for alternative medicine, and stick to this list when you are searching for remedies

Some people don't like to use anything that has been processed at all. Some people turn to essential oils for everything. Others don't like to use things they have to ingest, but others only like to use things they can take like modern medicine.

When it comes to your own personal care, you have to find what works for you, and go with that. No one can tell you that you're doing it wrong if you are happy with how it's going, and no one can tell you that you need to change the method you are using if you find that it works for you.

Lesson 16. Don't be afraid to keep your methods to yourself... unless you are with people who agree with your methods, you are going to end up with criticism

All in all, it doesn't really matter what other people say, but you are going to have to understand that this is a highly debated topic. While there are all kinds of real and true benefits so many people are so stuck in the way of thinking they are already in that they aren't open to any other ideas.

You have to be understanding as you go into this style of living that it's going to have you're going to have your supporters and you are going to have people that don't understand, but that doesn't mean it's not going to work.

Stick with it and you'll get the benefits... all without any modern medicine.

Chapter 5 – Alternative Medicine for Life

There is so much more to alternative medicine than just when you get sick or are feeling under the weather. This is a lifestyle that you can live out whether you are feeling poorly or not.

A large part of this lifestyle is healthy living in general. This is what is going to keep you going strong in your day to day life. Of course, everyone gets sick from time to time, but that's going to happen a lot less when you are living the alternative medicine lifestyle.

For the last few lessons, you have to develop this lifestyle in your life, so you are keeping yourself from getting sick in the first place. Of course, you are still going to have your good days and bad, but they are going to happen less frequently, and they aren't going to be as bad when they do happen.

Lesson 17. Learn to live a life of prevention... it makes the cure so much easier

Get in the habit of cutting out refined foods from your diet. Cut out all the processed foods, and try to cut out as many sweeteners as you can. I know it can be hard to get into this way of eating, but trust me, the more you get used to it, the less time you are going to spend sick, and the better your quality of life is going to be all around.

Of course, this doesn't mean you have to cut out all the sweets in your diet, but try to cut out most of them.

Lesson 18. Start to take measures as soon as you feel yourself starting to feel under the weather

For example:

We all know when we have that first twinge of feeling poorly. That moment when you suddenly feel like you could be getting sick... yeah, you know the feeling.

When that happens, it's time to kick your preventative measures into high gear. As soon as you start feeling yourself starting to get sick, cut out all the processed foods, cut out sweeteners, and make sure you are taking care of yourself.

Get to sleep on time, and make sure your quality of sleep is as high as it can be. Start to take your apple cider vinegar regularly. These are the active measures you can take during your alternative medicine.

Lesson 19. Understand your limitations

No matter what kind of lifestyle you live, there are going to be times you just need to sit back and relax. When you are using alternative medicine, you have to remember that there are days when you need to simply relax and let your body get some rest.

Remember to live your healthy lifestyle, and make sure you are eating right. The more you take care of yourself, the easier it is for you to stay healthy. All in all, you don't need to worry too much about what you are going to do if you fall sick, you just need to focus on living the healthy lifestyle and the rest is going to take care of itself.

Lesson 20. Be mindful of the pills you take, and remember that not all pills are bad. There are all kinds of pills that are made out of completely natural things and can be considered a part of the alternative medicine

If you simply browse the supplement section of any department store, you are going to find row after row of supplements from all kinds of natural sources. Whether you are looking for something that is plant based, minerals, or vitamins, you are going to find what you need.

There is some debate on what you can use in an alternative medicine lifestyle, but at the end of the day, what matters is how you feel about it. If you want to use supplements and minerals, use them!

If you want to stick to just produce and vitamins through food sources, do that. If you want to eat just like you always do, but you want to use methods such as aromatherapy, sound therapy, massage therapy, or anything like that, do it!

The biggest benefit to this life is that you can pick what it is you want to do, and you can base what you do on how you feel. I know there can be some confusion and question at first, but with practice, you are going to know exactly what you need to do.

The most important thing you have to remember is that it's ok to have other people disagree with you, and there are going to be times when they do. Simply stick with what you like to do, and do what feels the best for you. You are going to figure out what works right for you, and what you want to do long term.

The more you do this, the easier it is going to become, and the more you will be able to prevent illness from taking hold of you in the first place. The alternative medicine lifestyle is definitely one you have to get used to, but once you do, you aren't ever going to want to go back to doing things the other way.

The natural life is the good life, and it's going to give you the best benefits... for life.

Conclusion

There you have it, everything you need to know to get you started on the path to natural medication, and how you can use that all-natural medication to keep your life running smoothly.

I know when you first look at the list of alternative medications, you have to think that there's no way these things are going to really help you stay healthy, but they do. Countless cultures across the globe have all used alternative medication for hundreds of years, and with good reason.

You don't have to worry about side effects, you don't have to worry about the expensive doctor visits or outrageous medication prices, and you don't have to worry about standing in line with all the sick people at a pharmacy, waiting for your prescription to be filled.

With natural remedies, you are going to change your own life in a way like never before. Say hello to the all-natural way of doing things, and forget about all of the nasty side effects that come with synthetics.

I am going to change the way you view medication and your livelihood, and show you how to use the world around you for the greatest health benefits. Let this book transform the way you think about modern medicine and take you back into the world of alternatives, and reap all of the excellent benefits that come with it.

This book is meant to inspire and transform, and change your life for the better. Let me show you a new way of doing things, and open the door to a healthier you.

FREE Bonus Reminder

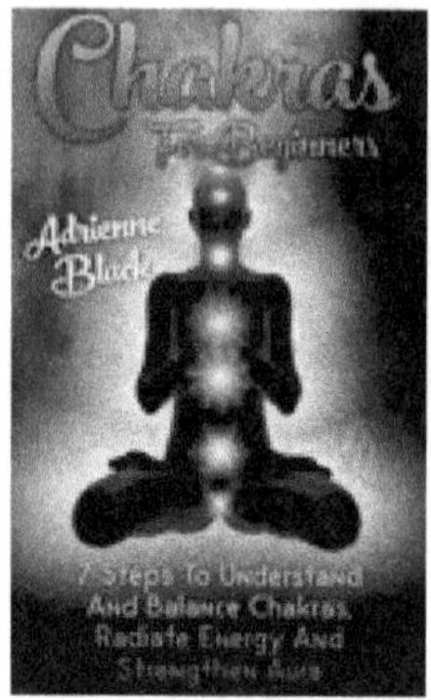

If you have not grabbed it yet, please go ahead and download your special bonus E book *"Chakras for Beginners. 7 Steps To Understand And Balance Chakras, Radiate Energy, And Strengthen Aura"*.

Simply Click the Button Below

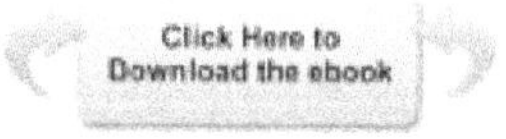

OR Go to This Page

http://lifehacksworld.com/free

BONUS #2: More Free & Discounted Books & Products

Do you want to receive more Free/Discounted Books or Products?

We have a mailing list where we send out our new Books or Products when they go free or with a discount on Amazon. Click on the link below to sign up for Free & Discount Book & Product Promotions.

=> **Sign Up for Free & Discount Book & Product Promotions** <=

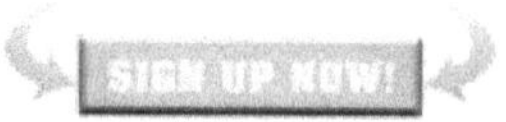

OR Go to this URL

http://zbit.ly/1WBb1Ek

www.ingramcontent.com/pod-product-compliance
Lightning Source LLC
Chambersburg PA
CBHW050806240726
48654CB00008B/649